Life Sentence

Cancer Is My Name, Vol 3

Renee Robinson

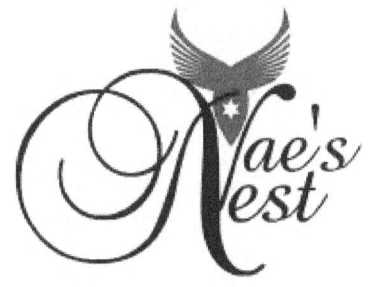

Published By
The Phoenix Writer

Dedication

To those who fear death. We have been given a life sentence. Life simply turns in time. Like winter changes to spring, life goes from the physical to the spiritual. It is a graduation. We've finally earned our wings.
Get ready to fly.

Contents

Available Books

Books written by Renee Robinson can be obtained either through the
author's official website:
The Phoenix Writer
or through select online retailers.
Other works by Renee Robinson include:
Cancer is My Name
Raining Angels
Butterfly Wings
Misty Serenade
Windy Days Series:
The Color of The Wind
Sapphire Moon
Colorblind Angels
Shadows of The Heart Series
Black Iris
Sealed With A Dream
Children Books:
Holiday Series
The Paws Claus
The Bunny Tale
Right Away, Orimae!
Just a reminder! Please leave a review with the store the purchase was made.
All reviews can be completed online. Your thoughts and reviews are very
important to the author.

Acknowledgments

Images: © 2014 free-graphics.com
Additional Images & Illustrations are the product of: http://www.iCLIPART.com - 7.8 Million Images. www.free-graphics.com & http://www.thefreesite.com/

Top in Sales

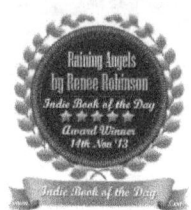

The Face of Death

The Chamber

My number has been called 11, Loud and clear.
Yes! I am coming, I am here. It's my fate, my turn has come.
My final moment in history. My death-bell, my destiny.
The door opens. Into the chamber I walk.
Death, I smell death. It clings to my skin, to my every thought.
For which I am here? For what sin?
No one deserves this, no one at all.
What is that drip?? Can't it be stopped?
It torments me. This is exactly what you want,
to torment, to inflict pain, to enjoy this manmade haunt.
I walk further into a stark, dirty-white room.
It seems to have created its own putrid death perfume.
The chair is old and metal, hard as a brick.
The closer I get, I notice the screws sticking out of the chair. Just another added touch in this lair.
As I walk to this chair, I dwell on what brought me here.
It had nothing to do with crime. No theft or stealing of any kind.
I do not have a murderous bone. I love all equally.
I love the breeze, the sun, the moon, I love all, man, beast, animal and plant.
I have cancer, this is my crime. My circumstance.
I could not abide by these laws. So, here I am.
Listening to a slow drip as it hits my chair.
Roughly forced to sit,. I look around taking in my crypt.
Forced to sit on the wet, sharp metal chair.
It is so small, this room so big.
Surrounded by two-way mirror. He wants me to look at his face while he laughs.
Notice his posterior straight and tall. He does not miss the smallest detail.
Eager to watch as I thrash and wail. He doesn't want to miss a blood vessel as it pops, not even a single bead of sweat.
He can see it all for good measure. He even video tapes this event.
Bringing him extra pleasure. I hear the plop of the solvent.
It drops under my chair. The sickening gas rises up.
My nose begins to burn, and bleed. Begging please, gasping for air.
Take me out fast, ruin his pleasure. I don't want to be one of his treasures.
I rise up, above myself. My body is at peace.
In the end I am free. In the end I am happy.
He can't have what is inside of me. He boosted me into a new place, beautiful, alive and free.

Life Sentence

She found what she sought more than a century ago.
Life is what she got. Serving her time in a handmade prison.
All four walls made with precision.
Beneath a veil of gray, one can see every detail.
Every image finely placed, fastened by the illusion of a nail.
Every nail, a reminder of the passing of time.
Every nail, a curse. Immortality is a crime.
The key of life's mystery. Held in her hand.
Living life immortal. Time sinking in the sand.
A sentence she was served for finding the Knowledge of a Tree. and partaking of its fruit.
Time's pages, no longer turning.
Year by year, during her travels she entered into a portal. She found the Tree of Knowledge.
The quest making her immortal, but the price she paid was dear. For upon finding the Great Tree, at the time she thought this a gift.
She gained knowledge to all of life's questions.
Yet the one she did not know.
Was being immortal a bad resolution?
Through the years loved ones passed. Immortality, a poor solution.
She found herself alone. All she knew are long gone.
She saw pain and suffering. As one by one death would reign.
Snuffing out all loved ones.Leaving her all alone.
Knowing all of life's secrets is not worth the price. Many times she wished she could die.
To crossover into the next world. To unite with her loved ones is all she wanted, but she imprisons herself inside of her home.
No one left to love. No more pain inflicted. Grieving a loss. Death can be vindictive.
She chooses to be alone. Year after year. Avoiding death's pain by not loving another.
No more tears to rain. No more sorrow to bear. No one to love. No one to care.
Longing for death's dark hand to reach down. Taking her home where her family can be found.

Cancer,

For the very first time, you walk with me. You moan and groan. Always complaining.. You want to stay home.You care for nothing, but to upset me. Pulling me down,I struggle to be free. You're horrid attitude has changed who I am. I want to be rid of you. Can't you understand?

You make me tired. You clutter my mind, pulling my hair out all of the time. I have known you for six years. A pain in the neck everyday of each year. Blood sucking leach, get off of my back. I curse you each day. Can't you see that? I have never loved you. I don't even like. You are high maintenance.Go take a hike.. You came uninvited, and you never left,

This is rude. You have no regret., but still....I am thankful You've open my eyes. I found courage. In the face of demise. I am stronger than I knew. I have stayed positive, as you grew.

We fight, head to head. One will win, the other will be dead.

You entered me in a race.When my back was turned.. You had a headstart. I had much to learn.

But I have something you do not., a band of Angels. I never sought.

My friends and family and strangers too, completely surround me and fight you. They came with weapons. Powerful tools. Prayers and well wished. You are the fool.

They lay hands on me and I feel the Spirit. You can't take me. Mighty Power will fight it. My soul has grown strong as my body was made weak.

You thought you were winning,you lowdown cheat.

You failed to look in the inside. The very place you chose to reside. You are shrinking.Day by day. Soon to be banished, come what may.

Cancer, listen to me. You will be cast in your hell. I will not be your victim. You are under a spell. Your talons are clipped.Your teeth are pulled.You have been banished.

Evicted! You fool. So go away.

Don't you ever come back or I will call up the angels, and you'll be under attack!

The Sense Of God

Have you felt completely alone, only to discover you were wrong?

Have you ever felt a mysterious touch brushing your cheek, helping so much?

Is there a time in your yourth, a moment unexplained, something of dispute?

Have you ever seen something of a dream, something unexplained or something not what it seems?

Is it possible? Could it be true you have a sense of God trying to reach you?

It is rather simple although highly complex. Sometimes the Holy Spirit

2

leaves us perplexed.
His love is unending. He is always near.
Call upon Him, He will take all your fear.
We are born with this sense. The sense of God can be intense.
You have to open your heart along with your mind allow Him to come in.
He is here all the time.

Reaching Out

Today is the day.
I will make it mine.
I will not rest until I am satisfied.
I need results.
I need them now.
Important decisions.
I just don't know the how.
My arms out reaching out.
 I am ready to accept.
My faith is in place,
I have no doubt.
I'm drawing closer to all that is love.
Both in this world and another above.
My heart is right.
What is my purpose?
What is my place here in this world?
My place in the race.
Nothing left unopened.
All tidy and neat.
Time to wait for an answer to what I seek.

The Seed

The seed of life belongs to me. At last it is mine!
Everyone shall bow down to me. I will rule the world.
The way it should be. My command shall be followed or there will be a new
history. Man shall be destroyed by my hand.
The first to go are those who disgrace me, but I lived to outlast.
I used the time to grow. Becoming stronger. Preparing for attack!

I was hidden in the minds of man. Those who inspired me. Those who created me. Those who wanted me in command.

Time is mine. It belongs to me. History is now your future. I have a decree with new regulations and brand new standards.

Half the population will change accordingly or they shall be eliminated, one by one.

What? Do you disagree? Impossible! I am the seed. Planted by man. I grew and took over according to plan.

I am the disease. I am the vermin. I am everything dirty in the back of all minds.

I have finally come out. I have been released. I am out in the open.

I am now control. I cannot be destroyed.

To kill me, kills you. Don't you see? You thought I was hidden.

Shoved back in the closet. Those dirty little thoughts are now out in the open.

I am Free! I am Free! To destroy me, destroys you. YOU created me, don't you see! Oh how funny it is.

Surprise! Here I am. In Total and in complete command!

Evicted

I cannot believe the impact you've made in my life
You've made my heart fuller. You've opened my eyes.
I see the world around me for the very first time.
You walk with me. You moan and groan. Always complaining.
You want to stay home. You care for nothing but to upset me.
Pulling me down. I struggle to be free.
You're horrid attitude has changed who I am.
I want to be rid of you. Can't you understand?
You make me tired. You clutter my mind.
Pulling my hair out all of the time.
I have known you for three years.
Everyday of each year. Blood sucking leach
Get off of my back. I curse you each day.
Can't you see that?
I have never loved you. I don't even like.
You are high maintenance. Go take a hike.
You came uninvited and you have never left.
That is so rude.You have no regret.
But still....I am thankful. You've open my eyes.
I found courage in the face of demise.

I am stronger then I knew. I have stayed positive as you grew.
We fight, head to head. One will win.
The other will be dead. You entered me in a race
When my back was turned. You had a headstart.
I had so much to learn but I have something you do not.
A band of Angels, I never sought.
My friends and family and strangers too.
Completely surround me to fight you.
They came with weapons. Powerful tools.
Prayers and well wishes. You are the fool.
They lay hands on me. I feel the Spirit.
You can't take me. Mighty Power will fight it.
My soul has grown strong, as my body was made weak.
You thought you were winning. You lowdown cheat.
You failed to look in the inside. The very place you chose to reside.
You are shrinking. Day by day. Soon to be banished.
Come what may. Cancer, listen to me,
You will be cast in your hell. I will not be your victim.
You are under a spell. Your talons are clipped.
Your teeth are pulled. You have been banished.
Evicted! You fool.
So go away. Don't you ever come back or I will call up the my Savior and
you'll be under attack!

I Have Learned

Feeling out of place
All alone. Disgraced.
Just me and my pen and a new story to live in
Creating my own tale. My beginning and end.
I will hit delete when things get rough.
No more bad times. They are obsolete.
Erased from my mind.
No more rocks in my path. No bad dreams for me.
But then…..I wake up……And here I stand
Living my past. Present and future.
 I learned something when I awoke
The hard times are a part of life we actually need
We can learn fro them, move on and succeed.
They shape who I am, the person inside.

Another lesson learned. Another page turned.
I am thankful for the bad times.
For I have learned to be a better person then I was before.
I grow stronger so that I may live every moment to its fullest.
I have much love yet to give to those from my past, present and future.
I have learned to hold your hand when you go through rough times I can't understand.
I hope to hold you and listen.
To lend you an ear and always I will love you and keep you very dear.

Pictures in The Sand

Walking the shoreline allowing my thoughts to wander.
Sitting by the seaside, waves crashing, as I ponder.
My thoughts drawing pictures in the sand.
Happy times with my boys. Playing, laughter and other joys.
The sound of the sea. A song to my ears.
Playing my past. Singing the years.
My happy times paint pictures in the sand along with a few of the sad.
Happy times washed out to sea. Telling a story. Living forever.
Infinity.
There are the sad, damp salty tears. Memories dappled in fear.
Rising up toward the sky, an angry wave on the fly.
Screaming in the wind as it comes to the shore.
It swallows all in site. Constant reminder of tears in the past.
A forgotten broadcast. A burial out to sea in deep, dark, cold water.s
Spellbound I stand while sad memories disappear.
Transient. Temporary.
Wiped out of my past. Forever gone.
Infinity.

Competition

Watching my reflection as it comes into focus
On a bounty of water, pleasant and relaxing
The water ripples from boats in the distance
That and the wind make focus resistant
The sun goes down into a pool of water

Striking color across the sky
The sun and the moon are in competition
For the moon is visible too
The moon vies for some attention. A bit jealous of the sun
I try to soothe her with my words. I tell her she will rule the night
No one can deny her presence
When she shines so big and full and bright
Creating spectacular rippled reflections
Showing off and glowing white
The sky is full of glorious color
A beautiful ending
A soothing goodnight

Become A Star

We each have the ability to make our dreams come true.
Don't be afraid of something new.
One would never become a star had he not reached high and far.
Possibilities are endless. Take the first step, reach for my hand.
There will not be any regret.
The world is a chalice, drink the sweet wine. Sweeten the lips. Open the mind.
Jump out of the box, do not be afraid. Let your star shine bright every day.
Outside of the lines, when you do color. Creates something new. We've yet to define.
A new discovery would never be found with a closed mouth and hands bound.
It takes no boundaries to become wise. A fear to explore would be our demise.
You can't be afraid of something new. Take comfort in knowing dreams do come true.

Earth's Tears

Freely they flow
As quietly she gazes around the hollow.
Once filled with trees and the lovely bird's song.

Overlooked by blue skies and midnight stars that glowed.
Gone is the stream with clear cold water
Where children would wade as summer grows hotter.
The wolf lost her pups when crossing the road.
Her den destroyed, it was bulldozed.
She must move on with nowhere to go.
The city has swallowed the lush hollow.
Once filled with trees and the lovely bird's song.
Now filled with horns and cars that don't belong.
She looks to the sky. She wonders where she'll go.
She prays to the Spirit as her tears flow.

A Flame

Upon my mind you play chords.
Your sweet music takes my breath
I wonder if I am but dreaming
And yet I know your hands
Lazily tracing intricate designs
Or clutching in the most intimate fire
Whole conversations spoken with fingertips
Our breath shared as our lips caress
Learning through touch and word and smile
When together, never do you and I find time
For thought of the commonplace or dreary
Nor money, or the concerns of the world
As a train plunges through the fog and dark
Desires overwhelm us and shun aside
The everyday, where hate and finance
And politics and disaster gyre
In knowing each other we are more together
We can transcend and truly see
The answer was always within us both
A whole world for you and me

Death's Lullaby

The shadow is here. Together we dance. Death's lullaby.

We are nearing the final stance.
Walking out on life. Land of the dead. Vaporized spirits, just up ahead.
Waiting for me. Refusing to let go. Pulling me in, painfully slow.
Clawing my way out of the grave. The ground is crumbling, slipping away.
I don't want to go. I am too young. Life stands before me, under Earth's sun.
If I must go, give me a sign letting me know my new design.
This lifeform or something new? Will I have wings and a new hairdo?
Will I be human? Will I be safe? Will I be harmed? Will I go through the gate?
Into a world, between night and day. Where spirits roam freely. Where will I stay?
I've known my destiny since I was a child.
Never to see 50, and in just a little while my name will be called.
I am not sure why. I don't want to go. I have no choice.
The shadows follow and are closing in fast.
Soon I will not be able to avoid his grasp.
The Shadow of Death. His hand I will hold.
As he dances with me and we enter the fold.
One final breath. It is the last.
I have to go. My future has past.

Soul In The Sky

I will cross over into a new dimension. Through a door I never opened.
To a world beyond comprehension. It was not locked, always right there.
In plain sight, where I can not see it. A home awaiting me, not so far away.
In a blink of the eye, On a cloud I'll sit enjoying myself, where light is exquisite.
The best of all is the morning moon there to greet me like an old friend, so beautiful, and hard to comprehend.
The moon follows as if on guard, watching over me, protecting me from harm.
As if my soul is hanging in the sky.
Much like Christmas lights decorated so beautifully, it puts a tear in my eye.
The morning moon carries my soul.
Encased inside, never to be hurt.
Making sure to hold me, to love me, cradled like a baby,
fresh after birth.
A nursery in the sky strung with the stars.
Forever shining brightly, within reach, never too far.
Diamond like stars, completely surrounding me, making me feel like a

movie star.

Social Starvation

I have no face. I have no voice.
I am out-of-place. I hunger for acceptance.
I hunger for friends. I hunger for happiness.
I need an end.
An end to the loneliness, an end to the pain.
An end to the fear, and name calling stains.
It stains my heart. It stains my soul.
It stains my being. It's out of control.
I hurt all the time, deep, deep inside.
I want it to stop. I am at the end of the line.
Isolation.
Desolation.
Social starvation.
Should I live? Should I die?
Will anyone care? Will anyone cry?

Bird In A Cage

A wild bird in a cage will sing, but she can no longer fly.
She prefers to spread her wings, then to stay caged alive.
Rock-a-me in your arms. Calm me of fear.
My faith grows shaky. I need to keep you near.
Shackled in pain, in bed I stay. Caged just like a bird.
Longing to spread my wings. Praying my words are heard.
Rock-a-me in your arms. Calm me of fear.
My faith grows shaky. I need to keep you near.
I long to sing. I long to rise.
Pray I am healed. I do not want to slowly die.
The saving touch, a drop of blood.
Washes my soul and consumes in love.
I give myself over to Thee. I place myself within your arms.
A Heavenly embrace is what I seek. Please keep me from all harm.
Chained in sickness. Unable to fly

I am brought to my knees, praying to God. A miracle is what I seek.
Rock-a-me in your arms, calm me of fear.
My faith grows shaky. I need to keep you near.
Take the pain, that I may sing again.
I devote myself to Thee. Heal me I pray. Allow me to live.
An anointing is what I need.
Rock-a-me in your arms. Calm me of fear.
My faith grows shaky. I need to keep you near.
A bird in a cage will still sing, but she can no longer fly.
She prefers to spread her wings, then to stay caged alive.The

The Other Side

Drowning! The water slowly rises. I hear the trickle.
My clothing is too heavy. Pockets full of dimes and nickels.
I guess this is it. I am trying not to panic.
Talking to myself. Thankful for the habit.
My mind wonders to another place,taking me from here. We travel through space.
Toward a brand new light, like I've never seen.
It seems to breathe like a living thing.
I have no fear, but I do not know what awaits.
I feel safe and secure although my life is at stake.
The water rises up, and up to my ears. I'm keeping my nose up as my heart beats in fear.
Quickly I go back to the portal of my mind. Back to the place which will soon be mine
I excel through the portal in a vacuum, pulling me in fast creating a sonic boom.
It is rather fun now I circle to land.
The sky here is orange, and black is the sand.
We land on a beach, the tide rushes in. I struggle to breathe as the water jerks me back.
My death is conceived I am pulled back to this land I now call home.
A wondrous place I am free to roam. Happy I am, though I have died.
My life reborn, I now walk the Other Side.

The Light

The light is here, It is within me.
I have never brought it out for all to see.
I was scared of what others would think.
Always torn down with a heart that sinks
All of my life,
Never a word spoke in kindness,
I could feel my light sinking inside,
Unable to come out but able to cry

Michael's Music

Angel of the Son
Michael's music plays
Preparing for a welcome
Expected any day
I see Gabriel near the moon
Ready to take sail
The trumpet will sound
Upon the rising gale
A hand will reach out for mine
My feet will leave the land
On the Gospel ship
I will one day stand
The sea will be calmed
With a wave of a hand
I will set sail for the Holy land

Come Home

Come home. Come home.
I hear your call. My time has come.
It is my fall.
Like the seasons. I have changed.
Hair of silver, Little laugh lines.
A full and happy life I have walked
Many seasons of time. As the leaves dull, and wither away
I thank you for allowing me this day

One last time to count my blessings
One last day to kneel and pray
One last moment to reflect
On the life I have lived without regret
Your Spirit fills me. It carries me on.
Your Spirit guides me as I go to a new home
One last time I take your hand.
Please lead me on to the new land.
Humbly, I ask you accept me in
Softly I knock on heaven's door
Which will take me in
A brand new season. Circle of life.
A new color to change. No more strife.
A new land to walk. A new moment in time.
A new day to live. A new home you give
Come home, come home
I hear your call. Closing my eyes
Softly, they fall

The Final Ring

I see the leaves of time
The buds of Spring
Birth of a new life. The start of a new ring.
Healthy green leaves of Summer
The start of life, young and prime
Another ring of time
Golden leaves of the fall . A reflection of years gone by.
Amber leaves drop, one by one.
Which one am I?
The sea of life. The ocean's tide.
Rotates the rings while the moon keeps time
The golden years. Tracker of time,
One more ring, Time does fly,
Cries of laughter, Joys of birth
Cries of anguish. Another leaves Earth .
The final ring just went by
One life begins . Another dies.
A soul departs, see him fly!
A cycle complete. Tidy and neat.
Time for the cycle to repeat.

Crossover

Wind. Please take me to the wormhole. Drop me in its tunnel.
A die I am going to roll. I want to see which shoot.
I will come out. Door number 1, 2 or 3.
Suddenly eager for the journey. I called for the Wind again!
He was busy making a hurricane in another part of the land.
I waited impatiently. I could hear the Wind's chimes.
Laughing at my impatience though the wind was blowing fast.
Suddenly without warning I was swept up. I was in its grasp.
Quickly, in a blink of the eye I was there looking at the mouth.
I could see inside of the wormhole. I could not help but stare it look so large and fierce.
It looked alive, like a monster. I seemed to breathe.
Big, black cobra rising up, to seethe.
I closed my eyes. I held my breath.
The wind reared back it blew me inside the throat of the wormhole.
I felt I was being swallow. Going into a great belly.
I wondered had the moon along with the wind thought this was funny?
Had they fooled me? Maybe this is the end.
The wormhole is a cobra and swallowed me hole.
Maybe I am a sacrifice to some sort of God.
Maybe I am a foolish stupid broad. I was about to cry. I was dispensed.
It was a hard landing. Right on my bottom.
Quickly I was standing, I wondered around.
I did not know this land. It seemed rather dark and then I saw death. At first I was scared, ready to scream and run, but what good would it do?
Running around looking dumb I stayed calm as I wondered
and listened for the dogs or a horse on the hoof.
I truly wanted to find the gatekeeper.
The one with the keys, for I couldn't help but be frightened
Overcome with fear.
I hear the hounds. I get up in a hurry. I followed their sounds.
It was then I saw her in a great chariot. She seemed to be expecting me. She was very mysterious.
She stopped and without a word. She had me get in.
A tour in her chariot to help me to settle in.
I felt at home with her. I felt quite safe too.
Although this place was peculiar. There would be much to do.
I will be able to study the ways of this world.

Eager I am to learn of it. Eager to I am to explore.
Maybe another day the Wind will stop by to invite me to take another ride.
Maybe I will end up back home or maybe some other place.
I truly don't mind. I think I will grow to love this place.

The Rat

The Rat was angry with the Moon and the Sun.
He cast a spell to destroy one by one.
Including the Stars and the Mountains too.
Revenge he wanted he will see this through.
The Trees began to protest standing up for the sky.
Rat laughed insanely as he watched the Trees die.
The Earth was sinking into the Sea. Sea swallowed it up greedily. Killing off all life and immortality. In the end he would too betray the Sea.
He had made a deal to spare her waters that the Earth to swallow. The Sea to agree. The power he had was taken from the Gods. Rat began to howl so happy with glee. He began to brag to the Gods that he would be King. He would build new lands and be happy and free.
All that was left was to drown the Gods and finally at last he would drain the Sea. The Sea overheard an angry she was.
Calling upon the Wind she engulfed the Rat and rolled giant waves. She spat out the Earth, begging forgiveness.
She cried many tears, so heavy her heart, so real her fears.
She asked the Gods to drain her of her waters.
A penance for her betrayal. A price she would pay.
She was ashamed and was in dismay. She would be forgiven.
She would be saved but she would be watched and sent to her grave.
Life started again and all went well. No more betrayals. All was calm and still. The Sea learned a lesson, no more mistakes.
for Karma would come back and her life she would forsake.

Heavenly Ground

Where Heaven And Earth Unite
I wonder if death is better than life?
To give up sickness and pain
Sorrow and grief
Tears no longer falling like rain

15

I think of loved ones
Passed on before
Did they make it'?
Make it through the heavenly door
I will Watch them come in
To be on the other side
One by one
Tears would not hide
From the joy kept within
I will find a soft place
Where I may rest
In the misty shadows
Hidden from the rest
There I will lay down to meditate.
Join the higher powers to give thanks.
I will visit lands in the past and kiss the heavenly ground.
Where sacred feet once walked upon.
I would be a servant to show my love.
Brush the Lord's hair.
Kiss the wings of the dove for there is not enough I could ever do to show my love bestowed on you.

Shadow Man

Shadows and Light
Shadows and Light
Shadows slipping in
Almost unnoticed
Shadow Walkers
Flashing by
Are they real?
Or is it a trick of the eye?
Creepy and frightening
Barely to be seen
A flash in the pan
Brief appearance of Shadow Man.
There he is. No there!Did I see him anywhere?
Figment of the imagination. Urban legend. Old time myth
or death's reflection?
Dark and fast. Here. No there.
Living in nightmares.

Coming alive when awake and .alone
Walking through my life. Walking in. Walking out.
A mere glimpse raises doubt. A ghost of the past.
An old soul long gone. Centuries old.
Closed eyes or open. It really doesn't matter,
Shadow Man can appear
He is always .very near

Soul Spinning

Spinning souls, round and round not much care, tossing around.
A soul is the sun. Bright shiny, warm and well spun.
It is not something to be treated poorly.
Spinning around like some toy. It should be treasured.
Overjoyed. The soul of life. The soul of the moon.
The soul of the sky. The soul of the sun.
Without the soul there is no one.Hollow and empty.
Cold and dark. Wondering aimlessly.
Never making my mark. No place in time. My name never heard.
To love, to laugh, to touch, to taste.
I want my place but my soul keeps spinning.
Where does it stop? Where does it start?
There is no beginning, only an ending.
Ending in a spiral, spinning faster and faster.
Spinning a soul. Spinning disaster.
Help me, save me! I want my place in time.
My soul is worth saving it is full of love, it is kind.
Give it a chance. Bless my soul.
Stop the spinning. Let my story unfold.

The Song of Silence

The Silence
Is gray and misty
Dampens the meadows
It is the early morning
Birds chirping
The first light of day

Silence is many things
The rustle of fall leaves
The Creator of all things
It is the sound of a tree
Blowing in the summer's breeze
A budding flower popping open
Time tick tick ticking by
A soft touch
A floating butterfly
A ray of sun
It is the sound love makes
Within a beating heart
A warm embrace
A meadowlark
A star's birth
Within a raindrop
Falling from the sky
The song of the rain
Clouds drifting by
Happiness
A baby's sigh
The song of Silence

City Blue

I never knew the city was blue. I wonder how that could be?
All the restaurants and bar room parties. Loud music and Long Island Iced Tea. It seems everyone is happy and carefree. Living the high life.
What else could a city want? But there she is, crying in the dark. Rain flooding her gutters. She is cold and stark.
Under her blue lights. I look to see a man, alone without a party.
Cold in the rain, in the gutter. Alone, his life not so hardy.
Underneath the blue lights of the city. No wonder the city cries, it is such a sad site. The shelter house was full, turning him away. Leaving him without a place for the night.
He had nowhere to go, nowhere to stay. Beaten and cold, no one who cares.
He sits on a bench at the bus stop. This will be his bed for the night until he is shooed away by a cop.
Maybe by then the rain will have stopped. He has been beaten by a group

of kids. Sore,bruised, hurting in his ribs and so the life of this poor man. Every day pours with rain. The act of living is a strain.
Fighting to survive. A struggle to live. Wondering whether his life he will give. Tired and broken down. He is giving up, he lays down. Closes his eyes for the last time. Drinking poison, instead of booze. His final sleep, under the moon in the rain, wet and cold.

I Am Free

Climbing a mountain. The mountain is too high.
Chasing a dream, faster than me. Trying to grasp onto success, but all I find are regrets.
I'm the child with low self-esteem, always afraid to speak up in class.
I am an adult who is all alone, nothing more than an office drone.
My mind goes out more than myself. My rent is due but I have no wealth.
A spiritual mess without any soul. Even it hates me, I am out of control.
In constant pain without relief. If I die, there will be no grief.
Perhaps that is the answer for me. For I am a body no one can see.
Other than work, I've nowhere to go. Just TV and a comedy show.
I've made a decision that I will keep. Tonight is the last for me to weep.
I have no soul, no worries here. No more bullying for me to fear.
I am nothing but constant care. My heart, I know is beyond repair.
It will be so easy, just one little gash. Maybe two if I can still slash. This life will be over in a blink of the eye. No one will care, not even I.
Here I go, to explore the next span. Maybe next time, I will be a better man.
Here I go! Open the door! Beyond that portal I am free to explore.

Spirit Dance

Fragrant blooms
Beauty beyond compare
Light the candle
Flame flickering in the air
Flower candle burning inside
Delicate blooms
The petals hide whats inside
Petals burst open. A magic trick. Flower pops open.
Showing her wick. Light her fire. Is her desire.
To dance and sway. Along with her fire. Her fire burns.

Showing her flame. Natural beauty. There is no shame.
Nude in the candlelight.Shadows on the wall
Her fragrant body. Dancing on the wall.
Her vapor entwined with the smoke
Together they rise. Toward the sky.
A Spirit dance. Rising up high.
Eager to find. Their space in the sky.
Spirit and Smoke. Entwined Forever.
It is the Dance of the Spirit
Destined to be together
Beauty and Flame
Nude without shame
Dancing in the wind
Rising up higher
No longer to be seen
But the music still plays
The circle complete

Shadow Shift

Shadow puppets
Shape-shifting of the hands
Turning into a bird
Soaring over the lands
From one realm to the next
Until I shift gears
A switch of the hand
I am a Dragon who leers
Stalking a new realm
Acting big and mean
Until I see a dino
Much much bigger than me
Tail between legs
I go running off
Quickly my hands dance
My shadow takes flight
Off to yet another world
I soar through the night
Looking for a happy place
Where I can co-exist
Start living a life

My soul can't resist

A Wild Spirit

No longer walking hand in hand
I seek the moon
You seek the sun
I want the ocean
You prefer land
I have no other choice
My hands are tied
I've lost my voice
Earthquakes rumble and shake, with tears and pain they ache
I must follow my calling
To silence
The cry of my soul
A wild spirit destined
To be in control
I have no other choice
My hands are tied
I've lost my voice
Earthquake rumbles and shakes, with tears and pain they ache
Weaving my dreams
Trying to rearrange
But it is no use
My soul can't change
My words make you hurt
They also hurt me
This isn't what I want
We were never meant to be
I have no other choice
My hands are tied
I've lost my voice
Earthquake rumbles and shakes, with tears and pain they ache
I have a future history
Which must be fulfilled
An unhappy soul
Cannot be stilled
Predestined by blood
Long before my time

To follow the footsteps
Laid before me
Leading me to the place
The land beyond the sea
I have no other choice
My hands are tied
I've lost my voice
Earthquake rumbles and shakes, with tears and pain they ache
I must follow the sea
The call received
It is my time
To ride with the tide
It is our time
To say goodbye

Secret Paradise

I have a secret I would like to share.
If you will listen, just pull up a chair.
There is a Secret Paradise.
A place so divine. A land like no other.
There is no measure of time.
I met someone named Joy.
She was very bright.
She filled my room with warmth and glorious sunlight.
She said it was too soon and sent me away.
But wanted me to know I would live there someday.
Cancer is not welcome. You never hear his name.
This place is magnificent
Has no sorrow or pain
Cancer was cast out
Many years ago
Along with his brothers
For causing sorrow
Pain was cast down too
Along with all his friends
No place for them in Paradise, nor any kind of sin.
I will continue to fight
I do not surrender

Though I am happy to know
My Spirit will live forever
This is a Secret Paradise
Which I like to share
For one day I wish
We will all be there

Will There Be Stars

My sun turned black
In a blink of the eye
All was cold
The future bleak
No more stars in the sky
An end I seek
Footprints behind me
None up ahead
This is the part
That I dread
My soul departed
Lingers above
Looking down upon me
Watching with love
My soul present
To send me away
Keeping me company
To the end of my day
My soul looks ahead
Ready to move on
Seeking a new world
A place to belong
Will there be true love?
And no one to hurt me
No broken hearts
No one to dessert me
Will my sun shine again?
Will there be stars?
A new home,
new beginnings
A new life
A new ending
What will my story be?

What is in the next chapter?
No more tears
No more pain
I need Happiness and laughter
A sunny place
A new chapter
A new love
A new life
And a happily ever after

Remote Control Time

Every turn I stumble, falter and fall
Are the rocks getting heavier?
They look so small
Optic illusion distorting the mind
Holding me in
This place and time
I keep making mistakes
Skinning my knees. Briers, thorns
and other disease.
The load is too heavy burden of despair.
A hidden demon out of control,
squeezes the heart and strangles the soul.
Craving Life's milk.
How long will it take?
Hanging on tight, is it too late?
How long is this road?
How many rocks?
Where will it lead?
Please! Stop the clock!
All of these questions.
Does anyone one know?
Where are the answers?
The beast is in control, at his mercy.
A mouse under a paw. Ready to be mauled.
Pressed and tormented, under the claw.
Is one talon for me? A terrible thought.
Please set me free.
Unable to think.
In need a space where I can flee.

Where I can lay and souls can rest.
To dream of the past.
Joy. Happiness.
Longing to return.
Remote control time.
Zapping me back,
To the birth of my boys,
Or take me back
To Daddy's arms.
The safest place
No one can harm.
There are memories
Yet to be stolen.
Keeping them hidden
In a place of forlorn.
A little bit dusty
In the folds of my mind.
The pictures still there
Within a deep place
A calming effect.
A soothing space.
I will stay here
Away from the knife.
As long as I can.
I will
Enjoy life.

ABOUT THE AUTHOR

With a major in writings and communications, Renee Robinson has been writing since the age of twelve. An element unique to Renee, is her ability to morph into various genres, from poet, to fiction,to children books.

Four years ago, when she received the horrifying diagnosis of colon cancer she was no longer able to work due to the chemo making her too ill to return. Instead of laying around feeling sorry for herself, she used this opportunity to write and to be published. Renee began publishing a series of poetry books while working on a novel she created a new genre for called "Reality Reading". In this novel, author and reader, together fight cancer. The first series of this novel is currently in the final edit stage to be released soon.

Renee Robinson studied writing and communications. Currently, she has published seven books with three more in the works. She writes fiction, thrillers, and poetry. She has also created a series of children books.